GETTING

SHREDDED

IS SIMPLE

HOW TO TRANSFORM YOUR BODY QUICKLY WITH COMMON SENSE

PAUL MAXWELL

OTHER BOOKS BY

PAUL MAXWELL

FINALLY FIT: BEAT LAZINESS, GET UNSTUCK, AND FINALLY MAKE YOUR GOALS STICK

GET IT ON AMAZON:
HTTPS://AMZN.TO/2Q5PFE7

ONE MORE TRY: WHY YOU ALWAYS FAIL AT FITNESS AND HOW TO FINALLY SUCCEED

GET IT ON AMAZON:
HTTPS://AMZN.TO/32WCBT2

AVAILABLE ON AMAZON

THEO.FIT

For discipline hacks & Fitness tips visit www.Theo.fit

Content

SECTION 3: CARDIO

SECTION 4: BASICS

SECTION 5: DIET

SECTION 6: IMAGE

SECTION 7: PERSPECTIVE

You have a
superpower.
It's called
"free will."

Every time
you say
"I can't,"
it is a lie.

The only person who can
save you from being "stuck"
is you.

No online guru.
No coach.
No book.

Only you.

Intro

Eat less. Move more. It's that simple.

My Story

I had wanted a six pack my entire life. But I never really *had* a six pack. I was always *kind of* in good shape. But I was never *shredded*. I thought it was impossible.

I tried exercise plan after exercise plan, diet after diet, and they all made me a better athlete — but they didn't give me the ultimate physique I wanted: the one with glorious abs and tons of definition. It always left me flabby in the gut, the chest, and the shoulders. Then, in my late twenties, I got my dream job as an acquisitions editor at a publisher.

I started listening to podcasts, and got into one diet called "the ketogenic diet." Basically, it said, eat no carbs, and lots of fat, and your body will get into "fat burning mode," and you'll lose a ton of fat! This isn't a bad diet. But I didn't realize that when you're eating lots of fat, it's very easy to eat thousands of calories without realizing it.

Nevertheless, I followed the diet very strictly. Working 80-hour weeks, I knew I needed to eat healthy. This diet was my attempt to do that. But then ... 3 months later, I had gone from 210 pounds to 240 pounds. Good Lord, what happened? Did I gain 30 pounds of muscle and turn into Arnold Schwarzenegger thanks to the ketogenic diet? Sadly, no.

Quite the opposite, in fact. I had never been so fat in my life. For the first time ever, I could feel "rolls" in my neck. It was harder to put my seatbelt on. My "man boobs" were ... uh, boob-y-er. I didn't know what to do. Then, I went back to the basics.

What did Arnold do to get so ripped? What do bodybuilders do to get so lean? After lots of research, I was hanging by my last thread of motivation. I had enough energy to try one more diet. If this didn't work, I told myself, I'd just accept the fact that I was "getting older," and that my best days were behind me.

So, I tried one more diet. It was a 12-week program. The principles were very simple. I followed it closely, with only 2 or 3 minor slip-ups per week. I worked hard. The diet was hard to keep. It was bland and boring and grueling. But I pushed through.

12 weeks later, I couldn't believe what I saw in the mirror. Not only had I lost the fat I gained ...
I was in the best shape of my entire life. I actually had a six pack. I real, visible, abs-popping-

like-rolls-in-an-oven six pack. I went from 240 pounds to 190 in 12 weeks.

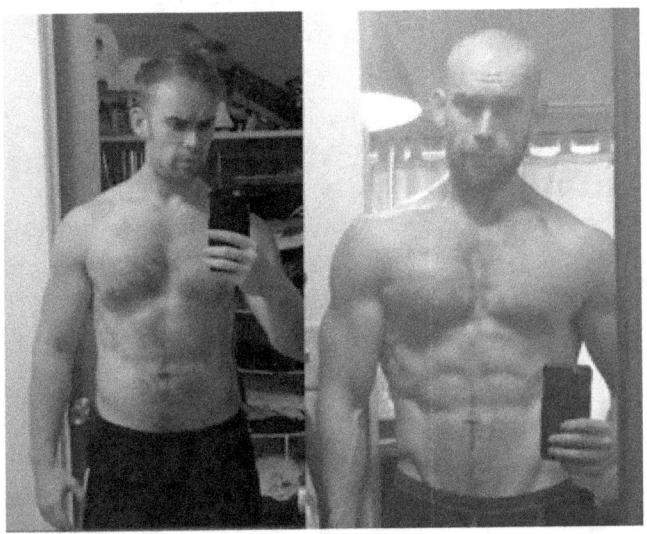

Was it unhealthy? Well, I actually gained muscle during that time, so I wasn't exactly "wasting away." I had found the holy grail of diets — the one that actually gave me the physique I wanted, and made me healthier at the same time!

I couldn't believe it. But then, I found something even more shocking. I tried to get my friends to do the diet — especially the ones who wanted to lose weight. And I was shocked at how nobody wanted to do it. Shocked. They all asked for my advice: "How did you do it, man?" And I told them. But here's the response I got from everyone:

"Actually, I did some research,
and I think I'm gonna
try something else."

Some just wanted to lift weights and run. Some wanted to try the high fat diet (the one that made me gain all the fat). Some wanted to try other little "tricks" and "hacks" and "plans" that had cool graphics and good marketing.

And guess what? None of them made any meaningful change in their physique. Not one. So I started a little fitness brand called *TheoFit*, and got a few people to do it with me.

The ones who adhered instantly dropped fat, and are still losing fat to this day. They're telling me: "I'm starting to look like I did in high school." They've started coaching other people. They, too, are shocked by how often people just want to try the "easiest plan" as opposed to the one that clearly works.

If you're tired of Googling "How To Get In Shape" every April, in desperate hope of getting in not-embarrassing shape for summer, follow these principles. Read this book. Make decisions to follow these guidelines in your life. And I guarantee, you will be amazed at what you see in 12 weeks — a person you haven't seen in a long time, possible ever: your most-fit self.

You can have the body you never thought was possible.

The beauty of these principles is that they're flexible. They work with calisthenics, running, weight lifting, whatever — they can bend to lots of different diets and exercise routines. That's why you should never fall for the Instagram Model's sales pitch that they have the "one piece" that stands between you and your six pack. I promise: It's in this book. It's common sense. You just need to be told what you already know.

The revolution you need to undergo in your thinking, if you're ever going to get in shape, is this:

> You have to stop asking "What?"
> and start asking "How much?"

Getting a six pack is not about "what" you eat or "what" exercises you do. Getting in shape is 100% about "How much" you eat, and "how much" you work out.

Stop trying to find the special "what" that's going to make your fat melt off — the answer isn't a special root, spice, carb ratio, or workout. Fat loss is 100% about how much you eat, and how much you work out — fat loss is about eating less, and moving more.

I wish it wasn't true. Maybe some day, centuries in the future, we will invent a "six pack pill." But for now, the only path to being shredded requires strict discipline. The only saving grace of this process is that it is so simple, and so within the reach of your willpower, that a kindergartener could explain it to you: eat less, move more.

The logistics of doing that can get complicated when we try to juggle that with our responsibilities. at's what this book is about — answering the most common reactions to "Eat Less. Move More." I get so many questions that start with "Yeah, but what about...?"

That's what this book is about. Charging the front line of mental and logistical obstacles in your battle against your flabby mid-center. I'll walk you through some of the initial difficulties that eating less and moving more can bring to your life.

Join with me. Getting ripped isn't easy. But it

is very simple. So let's stop making excuses, and start doing what we already know we need to do in order to get the bodies we never believed we could get.

1

How does a "Cut" help me to get in shape?

A "Cut" is when you lose as much fat as possible, while maintaining as much muscle as possible. A cut has three essential elements. If you compromise on one of these, you're going to end up skinny-fat, over-trained, or frustrated that you didn't meet your fitness goals. There are three essential elements of losing fat as fast as possible:

> (1) A 20% Calorie Deficit
> (2) Weight Lifting 5 Times a Week
> (3) 1 Gram of Protein per
> Pound of Bodyweight

(1) A 20% Calorie Deficit

What that means is, if you burn 2000 calories per day, you should be eating 1600. You could be running marathons every day, lifting for 3 hours, and eating only chicken and lettuce — but if you're not in a calorie deficit, you're not going to lose fat.

(2) Weight Lifting 5 Times a Week

If you don't lift weights while you're in a calorie deficit, you're just going to become a "smaller version" of your current self. Your fitness goal

There's no benifit to becoming smaller if you're remaining just as fat.

isn't to "lose weight," but to lose fat. There's no benefit to becoming smaller if you're remaining just as fat. Weight lifting is essential for ensuring that the weight you lose really is fat, rather than fat and muscle.

(3) 1 Gram of Protein per Pound of Bodyweight

You need to be eating 1 gram of protein for every pound of body weight. Some people say this is bogus — that humans actually need far less protein than we often think. This is true if you're not lifting weights, doing cardio, and in a calorie deficit.

If you're a sedentary person with no fitness aspirations — if you're not exercising while in a calorie deficit — then eat 50 grams of protein a day! It's not a big deal.

But if you're challenging your body to burn energy, and you're lifting weights, you need to give your body all the resources it needs to repair your muscles and maintain your strength while you're in a calorie deficit. Otherwise, your body will break your muscles down and use them as energy. You want something to show off beneath the fat when you lose it! That's why protein is important.

The Most Important Part of a Cut

Of these three elements — a calorie deficit, weight lifting, and protein — the calorie deficit is by far the most important. There are two ways to get into a calorie deficit:

> (1) Move more.
> (2) Eat less.

People will try to sell you all kinds of fitness routines:

> "Buy my custom meal plan!"
> "Buy my 12 week shredded program!"
> "Sign up to my email list to

get my 45-page PDF
that explains the key to getting ripped!"

It's all a B.S. way of stroking your ego and making you feel like you're missing some essential piece of information you didn't have before. But there's only one secret to losing fat:

Eat less.

It's a cruel world. The laws of physics don't respect our quest for a healthy body image. In order to lose fat, we simply have to be in a calorie deficit for a long period of time.

One pound of body fat = 3500 calories. If you're in a 500 calorie deficit every day, that means you'll lose a pound of fat per week. If you're in a 1,000 calorie deficit per day, you'll lose 2 pounds per week. It's that simple.

I'll explain how to do this effectively and intelligently throughout this book. But never forget this simple rule:

Don't try to outsmart your caloric consumption.

Your thyroid is never going to make a pound of fat = 10,000 calories.
What's your fitness goal? A six pack? Toned

The laws of physics don't respect your quest for a healthy body image.

arms? Losing the man boobs? Getting rid of the gut? Being happy to take your shirt off at the beach?

The answer is not The Whole 30. The answer is not "eating clean." The answer is not your jazzercise class. The answer is not bench pressing 300 pounds. The answer is not cutting caffeine. The answer is not cutting gluten. There is only one answer. Say it with me:

Calorie. Deficit.

The calorie deficit is the key to the cut. Lifting and protein are footnotes. Nail your 20% calorie deficit, and within 3 months, you will look like a completely different person. It's physics.

2

Is it possible to follow the rules of a "Cut" and not see results after 12 weeks?

If your goal is to lose fat — and losing fat is the key to getting toned, losing the gut, feeling healthier, etc. — then no, it's not possible to follow these three simple rules and not see results in 12 weeks.

If you're in a 20% calorie deficit, lifting, and eating one gram of protein per pound of body weight for 12 weeks, you will look and feel like a completely different person.

The real question is: What are you waiting for? Why aren't you starting this plan today? Why are you making so many excuses? Why are you telling yourself "I can't" when you obviously can, but just aren't willing to?

I'm giving you the script to a guaranteed revolution of your body. You have no excuses. Your current body is not my responsibility. It's not society's responsibility. It's your responsibility alone. These principles take different shape for everyone.

Find a way to stick to these rules that works for you. Don't B.S. yourself. Don't fall into the trap of thinking, "I tried that and it didn't work for me, so diets don't work." No. You didn't do it right. You didn't do it well. Get in your deficit. Get to the gym. Get your protein.

It's in your power to change your body.

Will you?

Envision yourself in 12 weeks.

Look at your calendar. What's the date today? What's the date 3 months from now? Is it May 15th? Imagine August 15th. You could have lost your gut by then.

You could have lost your love handles by then. You could have lost your chicken neck by then. You could be carrying 20-30 pounds less by then.

That makes getting up in the morning easier. That makes getting out of the car easier. That makes work easier. That makes walking easier.

That makes playing with your kids easier. That makes getting a date easier.

Will you do this, or not?

It's you vs. you. Imagine yourself today, in the mirror, side by side with you in 12 weeks, totally transformed. You're either going to become that person, or you're not. **Will you convince yourself "I can't" for the millionth time, or will you become that person you've always wanted to be for the first time?**

It's in your power to change your body. This book gives you all the knowledge you need. It's very little. Will you do it, or not? Your body is in your hands. Change yourself. You can do this. Make it happen.

3
Do I really have time for a cut?

You may be thinking:

"I'm going to ease into this whole 'getting in shape' thing. I'll work out a little bit. Jog a little more. Eat McDonald's a little less. But I'm not about to do 'a cut' — I'm not trying to be a bodybuilder here."

Let me respond to that voice.

First, a cut is probably easier than whatever you're going to do, except it is more informed, requires less time, and gets far better results. Second, I want you to be honest with yourself — have you ever, ever tried to get in shape and ended up with the results you wanted going into it?

In other words, have you ever succeeded in attaining your dream body? (You know, the one you wished you had in college)

For ten years I didn't accomplish my vision. I just gave up — I assumed that only fitness models with "insider knowledge" could get chiseled bodies and six packs. en, when I learned the right information, it took me 12 weeks. Six pack. Veins running across my abdomen, and in my arms.

Never had that before in my life. Never thought

Don't have time for a cut?

Guess what: Eating less food takes less time.

it was possible. Discovering the cut trifecta —
calorie deficit, weights, and protein — was like
discovering a cheat code to getting in shape.

Third, if you don't do a cut now, when are you
going to do it? Do your summer-self a favor.
Accomplish the body you want in 12 weeks. Don't
tell yourself "I don't have time." Guess what?
Eating less food actually takes less time.

Granted, preparing food that makes 1600
calories fill you up as if it were 2600 (like lots of
salads) can be more work than scarfing down a
bagel with cream cheese from Dunkin Donuts.

But we're talking minutes of time here. Not hours.

(Also: think of the extra years, possibly decades you'll be adding to your life in your 70s and 80s … that gift starts with habits formed today).

4
Will I really
see results?

In other words:

> Is it possible to (1) have a 20% calorie
> deficit, (2) lift 5x5x5 3-5 times per week,
> and (3) consume one gram of protein per
> pound of body weight, and not see results
> after 12 weeks?

No. So, if you're not seeing results, try lowering
the food intake or upping the exercise (cardio
is the most efficient way to burn calories, but
too much cardio can compromise your muscle
retention).

The biggest mistake in calculating your calorie
deficit is in assuming you burn more calories
than you really do.

When I started my cut for the first time, I ate
about 2600 calories per day as a 6'1" 240 male.
I didn't lose any fat for three weeks. So someone
told me to shoot for 2200. When I did, the fat
melted off over the next few weeks.

When you're calculating how many calories you
need to burn, it's always better to over-calculate
the calories in the food you eat, and under-
calculate the amount of calories you should be
consuming.

If, after two weeks of a calorie deficit, you're not losing fat, the solution is simple:

eat less or move

Again, a pound of fat = 3500 calories. Your daily calorie deficit is meant to accumulate so that over time, you lose pound after pound. The bigger your deficit, the faster you lose weight.

If, after your first two weeks, you're not losing a sufficient amount of fat, lower your daily calorie intake by 100 calories and adjust accordingly.
It is important to know what are your BMR and TDEE.

BMR = Basal Metabolic Rate = Calories burned per day, at rest.

TDEE = Total Daily Energy Expenditure = Total calories burned in a day, including exercise and daily activities.

5

Is there a simple way to calculate my calorie deficit?

The below chart is assuming you're performing resistance training 4-5 times per week—with about an hour of cardio per week. Based on generic principles, this is about what you should consume each day. To get a more specific calculation, visit the website below. But remember: it's always better to round down on your calorie deficit, not up. Otherwise, you're wasting your time.

The goal during a cut isn't to become strong or fast, but to lose fat. If your energy is low and you feel deflated, that's because you're consuming less energy (calories) than you're accustomed to. Don't fudge on your calorie deficit because you think you need to "fuel" your workouts. at's what your extra body fat is there for.

Weight (lbs)	BMR	TDEE*	30% Deficit	20% Deficit	10% Surplus
340	3200	3600	2520	2880	3960
320	3100	3500	2450	2800	3850
300	2900	3300	2310	2650	3630
280	2800	3200	2240	2560	3520
260	2700	3100	2170	2480	3410
240	2600	3000	2100	2400	3300
220	2400	2800	1960	2240	3080
200	2200	2600	1820	2080	2860
180	2000	2400	1680	1920	2640
160	1800	2200	1540	1760	2420
140	1700	2000	1400	1600	2200
120	1600	1800	1260	1440	1980

*Based on intense exercise 5-6 times per week.

6
When will I see results?

If you're adherent, you will see results. But I do understand the mania that this process can induce — constantly looking in the mirror, grabbing fat, hoping you can hate the fat so much, it will want to run away.

Here's the mindset you need to have during the first 6-8 weeks: *Don't look for results.* Yes, you should still weigh yourself — you need some way to measure progress so that you know if you need to increase your deficit (i.e., if you're not losing weight, you need to eat less). But nobody goes on a diet just to lose weight. We want to be healthier. We want to look better. And those are the results that we have to commit not to think about for the foreseeable future.

If we think too much about these results in the early stages of a cut, we will go insane. Commit to 6-8 weeks of slogging, bland, boring, grueling tasks. Misery? Yes. But the more miserable you make yourself with discipline now, the better the sooner you will see the results you're really after.

"Lean in" toward the misery — as long as it's informed, strategic, and consistent, none of it will be in vain. In a sense, you must "diet by faith" that the laws of physics will have their way with you, and that your body will oxidize your body fat for energy. If you follow the three principles of the cut, and you don't see drastic body changes in by weeks 10-12, you've entered an alternate universe.

39

Part 2

CALO RIES

7

Is a calorie deficit really healthy?

For a short period of time, yes. If you stay in a calorie deficit for long enough, you will starve to death. That's why people who are always "on a diet" are chronically unhealthy and fluctuating in their weight. They think it's better (to borrow from Ron Swanson) to half-ass a bunch of diets that don't work rather than whole-ass the one diet that does work.

People who chronically under-eat usually end up malnourished and weak, perhaps with a mild case of anorexia. Any diet that requires you to be in a calorie deficit for the rest of your life is trying to kill you.

The 12-week cut is perfect for people who love food, and want to restrict their diet for as short a time as possible. The more consistent you are with your 20% calorie deficit during your cut (perhaps going into 25% or 30% toward the end), the shorter you have to be in a calorie deficit!

The goal of a diet isn't to diet forever, but to lose fat, create a better-looking, healthier "normal" for your body, and get back to a well-nourishing, sustainable diet that gives your body everything it needs.

Unfortunately, in order to lose fat, you must be

If you are 100% adherent to the three principles, you will see fast and fulfilling results.

in a calorie deficit. It's not enough to "restrict calories." You have to actually figure out how many calories you burn in a day, and consume 20% fewer calories than that number for 12 weeks in a row.

The purpose of this is to "starve" your body for as short a time as possible. You want your body to have insufficient energy to run so that it uses your body fat for energy.

It doesn't matter what time you eat. It doesn't matter what kind of food you eat. It doesn't even matter if you get all your food from McDonald's. If you are in a calorie deficit, you will lose weight.

The goal is to be in a calorie deficit while maintaining as much strength as possible, so that the weight you use is fat.

How do you currently feel about your body? Do you wish you could get rid of fat rolls? Do you find that you're uncomfortable in your own skin? Do you wish you could weak your bathing suit to the beach and feel comfortable? Do you have trouble walking, or running, a mile?

If so, a calorie deficit paired with sufficient exercise and protein intake could be the healthiest thing you could possibly do.

Most people who develop chronic malnourishment from under-eating (1) aren't trying to maintain strength through weight lifting, or (2) have been in a calorie deficit for 6 months or more. Both of those are obvious ways to "waste away" into a bag of bones. at's just as unhealthy as obesity. Being "skinny" should never be the goal.

Getting lean, on the other hand, is a double-goal of pursuing strength and fat loss at the same time. If you currently have no sense of what to do to lose fat, begin here: the calorie deficit. Don't let your internal voice convince you that you're becoming

A calorie deficit is not unhealthy if it is strategic and purposeful.

"anorexic."

No. You love food. I love food. The goal is to cut as hard as we can for as short a time as possible so that we can return to a sustainable lifestyle with a better-looking, healthier body.

For you, a calorie deficit is not unhealthy. It's the most healthy thing you could possibly do for the next 12 weeks.

8
How do I count calories?

The first thing you need to do to count calories is download a calorie-counting app. The best two are My Fitness Pal and MyPlate. They are basically identical. It doesn't matter which you use. They each have a verified database of food's caloric value. These are 95% reliable.

Every single piece of food you eat counts — from a tab of butter, to the oil you use to cook your food, to the scone-piece you scrap from the office brunch party. Log everything you consume. Drinks. Condiments. Meals. Everything. Your fitness app will have the accurate caloric value. (If you don't have a smart phone, you can just use your computer to find website versions of these apps, or use a physical journal).

At the end of the day, your sum total caloric intake may surprise you. It's much harder to hit a caloric deficit than we think, largely because the foods we are accustomed to eating contain many more calories than we suppose.

For example, a peanut butter and jelly sandwich with 3 tablespoons of peanut butter (less than I usually use) and 2 tablespoons of jelly is 500 calories. A large garden salad with low-fat mozzarella cheese, low-calorie dressing, and a half-pound of grilled chicken is about 400 calories.

No matter what you eat, the important thing is to achieve a calorie deficit.

The sandwich is about a pound 0.25 pounds, and 1/8 of a gallon in volume. The salad is about 0.75 pounds, and 0.5 gallons in volume! That means the salad is fewer calories, but 3-4 times more filling. In other words, it would take 2,000 calories worth of PB&J to "fill" the same amount of space in your stomach as the salad.

So, when aiming for a calorie deficit, counting calories helps you to choose "bigger," but lower-calorie foods to fill you up, rather than "smaller" foods with the same calorie value that leave you feeling hungry (even if they taste better).
In summary, you count calories by logging them

in your phone's app. You stop eating when you hit your calorie limit for your day. at's all there is to it. It's easier said than done, but don't let anyone tell you it's more complex than that. Losing fat is 90% about eating fewer calories.

The adventure becomes finding out how to eat the most amount of food you can possibly eat within your calorie budget. Usually, high-calorie foods are tasty, but small and unsatisfying. When you're aiming for a deficit, try to make your food taste good in low-calorie ways. And make them as accessible as possible. For instance:

- Use spices and seasonings instead of sauces.
- Use lettuce (50 calories per head) instead of bread (100 calories per slice).
- Use low-fat alternatives of everything.
- Buy the "lean" meat (95/5, or 99/1) at the grocery store, instead of the "fat" meat (70/30). Lean meat is about half the calories, but tastes just as good.
- Use almond milk instead of dairy milk.
- Don't keep tempting foods in the house.
- Prepare your food ahead of time, and take it with you, so that you aren't caught without food near a fast food restaurant.

There are more tips we will explore later, but you can start here.

9

I keep going over my calorie limit. Any tips for hitting your deficit each day?

Yes. is is where things get a little more about what works for you, rather than "right" or "wrong" diet doctrine. For example, the only way I hit my calorie deficit each day is if I only eat one meal a day — dinner. Then, I'm full, and I can sleep.

Yes, I'm hungry throughout the day, but I know I'm going to have a hearty 1,800 calorie meal at night, so the hunger is more bearable. I am an "indulger."

Now take my wife Molly. If she tries to wait all day to eat, she gets tired, she gets headaches, she loses willpower. As a result, waiting all day to eat usually results in a high-calorie binge around 2:00pm.

Then, when she is hungry by dinner, she eats a modest meal, but goes way over her calorie goal. So, it works better for her to eat 5 smaller meals per day. Molly is a "grazer."

Like everything with fitness, the best habit is the one you can consistently keep. So, whatever you need to do to hit your calorie goal, do that. If you like eating a big breakfast and a small dinner, do it. If you're like me, and would rather pig out at night, do it.

The best diet is the one you can keep. As long as you hit a deficit, you're on the right track.

If you like to graze throughout the day, find the best times to eat that give you the most focus and energy, and eat at those times.

Pulling off a calorie deficit is no good if it makes you so miserable, you quit after a week. A calorie deficit will always be grueling to some degree. So don't think there's such a thing as an "easy deficit." Hunger is always hard. But. There are more sane ways of doing it, and less sane ways of doing it.

Besides meal timing, there is one other important tactic to keep in mind as you try to hit a calorie deficit that feels really hard:

Eat a lot of low-calorie foods.

For example, before I eat my big meal at night, I will eat three heads of Romaine lettuce within a 15-minute window, just so that the meal I eat will feel filling.

Another tactic similar to this is: eat a lot of low-calorie food right after your meal. For example, zero-sugar Jell-O is 10 calories per cup. Eat A GALLON'S WORTH of sugar-free Jell-O for 160 calories (by the way, that's about half a "Clif Bar"). Finding the sanity you need to hit your calorie deficit can often come down to a combination of will- power and guerrilla tactics for feeling full.

Find your favorite low-calorie food and use it as a crutch until your 12 weeks are over. And when you're tempted to indulge, to break your calorie deficit, always keep in mind: ***this is not forever.***

You're not relinquishing yourself to a life of starvation. A cut is a focused few weeks of restriction. Find your sanity in the fact that when it's over — and it will be soon — you will look and feel like a different person.

10

Can't I just "eat clean" instead of being in a calorie deficit?

Understand "Macros" and "Micros"
In order to understand the answer to this question, we have to understand the difference between macronutrients and micronutrients. Macronutrients ("Macros") are your Fats, Carbs, and Proteins. Micronutrients ("Micros") are vitamins and minerals, like Vitamin C and Iron.

"Clean eating" usually refers to eating food with lots of good micros. The problem is, to lose fat, you need to be in a calorie deficit, and you do that by eating less macros. In other words, you're not going to shed pounds by increasing your "vitamin-full foods" intake. If that was the case, multivitamin pills would be a miracle drug for fat loss.

Instead, weight loss happens from eating less macronutrients. Each micronutrient — fat, carbohydrate, and protein — has a different caloric value:

> 1 gram of carbohydrates =4 calories
> 1 gram of protein =4
> 1 gram of fat =9 calories

So, your calorie deficit all comes down to how many grams of carbohydrates, protein, and fat you consume. For example, 20g of protein is 80 calories. It doesn't matter if that protein is

> # *Some people lose weight on "clean eating" programs because they eat fewer calories by accident.*

in lardy bacon or lean egg whites. Food becomes high in calories when it contains more sugar and fat. e reason a cheeseburger is twice the calories of a chicken sandwich is because a cheeseburger is comprised more of fat than protein, and therefore more calories. A chicken breast is extremely lean, containing mostly protein, and is therefore much lower in calories.

Why "Clean Eating" Works (Sometimes)

So, you could eat Whole30 for a year, eat zero

carbs, cut gluten and dairy, eat only organic everything, and still end up gaining 30 pounds (a lot of people do) if you eat more calories than you expend. Some people lose weight on "clean eating" programs because they end up eating fewer calories by accident.

But when it comes to fat loss, eating fibrous sugar (like an organ) isn't objectively "better" than eating a Snickers bar, or an ice cream cone. At the end of the day, you're just as well off eating a Klondike Bar with a Vitamin C tablet as you are eating an orange. In fact, if you enjoy ice cream more than oranges, you're probably better off doing it.

Why Calorie Counting Works Better

However, "clean" foods usually don't taste as good, but they fill you up without a ton of calories. So, a mini pack of Oreos can be 300 calories, but a chicken salad can also be 300 calories. One tastes better, but the salad doesn't leave you feeling hungry, so it makes the calorie deficit easier. A study was done at Kansas State University where a nutrition professor ate twinkles and McDonald's, and lost 30 pounds in two months. How? He restricted his diet to 1,800 calories a day. at's it.

His study proves that any weight loss plan comes down to consuming fewer calories than you expend. In sum, "eating clean" is a good long-term strategy for health, and it helps you keep hunger at bay during your cut. Just don't confuse "eating clean" for "losing fat." You have to be in a calorie deficit to do that.

11

What are common "health foods" that easily ruin a calorie deficit?

Anyone who's seen the movie Mean Girls remembers the scene when the main character gives the bully girl a "weight loss" bar. The bully later discovers that the bar is actually a "weight gain" bar that the football team uses to put on pounds.

Sadly, the "Health Food" industry can play a similar trick on well-meaning dieters. Similar to a fitness center throwing a "pizza party" for its members, "health food" is meant to keep you eating its products, under the belief that you need them to be lean.

But remember: a cut isn't about becoming a "health food" person, but losing as much fat as possible in as short a time as possible. Don't get sucked into "health food" culture in your attempt to lose fat. It will, more often than not, keep you fat.

Here is a list of foods commonly thought to be "healthy," but will more than likely destroy your goal of losing fat by ruining your calorie deficit:

A cut isn't about becoming a "health food" person, but losing as much fat as quickly as possible.

"Health Food"	Caloric Value	Amount
Olive Oil	100	1 Tbsp
Egg	234	3 Eggs
Peanut butter	200	2 Tbsp
Strawberry Jelly	110	1 Tbsp
Whole Grain Bread	150	2 Slices
Avocado	330	1 Avocado
Raisins	129	1 Small Box
Grape Nuts	416	1 Cup
(w/ skim milk)	(506)	1 Cup
Salmon	354	6 oz.

Let's pause here for a second. Let's say this chart represents your daily eating habit. You cook your 3 eggs in a tablespoon of olive oil (don't be fooled by cooking spray — it does have calories). Then you have a light PB&J sandwich for lunch. A small salmon filet and an avocado for dinner. And a bowl of grape nuts for dinner.

That's 2,023 calories. If you're a 200 pound man, and you've exercised vigorously for an hour, you are not allowed to eat anymore, or else you will break your deficit.

> Small omelet.
> Small sandwich.
> Small fish filet w/ small side.
> Small bowl of cereal.
> That's it. Seems healthy, right?

What if we doubled lunch and our snack? What if we ate a regular-sized PB&J sandwiches, and a regular-sized (2-cup) bowl of grape nuts? en we'd be at 3,000 calories — now gaining fat. And that's just:
> Small omelet.
> A regular-sized PB&J sandwich.
> A small fish filet w/ small side.
> A regular-sized bowl of Grape Nuts.

This shouldn't cause us to despair. It's just a

warning: check the label. Make sure you're not eating a lot of something just because it's from Whole Foods.

"Healthy" is just a marketing company's way of getting you to buy their food. Just because the packaging looks like it was plucked straight from Farmer Joe's hands at an organic farm, doesn't mean it's low-calorie. Remember: the calorie deficit is the end game. Don't let the "health food" industry obscure that.

12

Why do I have to be in a calorie deficit to lose weight?

As we mentioned earlier:

1 pound of fat = 3,500 calories

Get Nerdy With Me

The body has two kinds of energy: glucose and ketones. Carbohydrates and proteins can be broken down into glucose. Fat is converted into ketones. Glucose is often referred to as our "fast energy." Ketones are slower- burning.

Now, for the all-important point: the word "calorie" is just a way to measure energy. The word "calorie" is just like the word "inch," or "minute." It's an arbitrary, but fixed, measurement. And we use the term "calorie" to refer to the energy in our bodies, in the form of glucose and ketones.

To summarize:

The body converts carbs and protein into glucose. The body converts fat into ketones. Both glucose and ketones are converted to calories.

Brief aside: The fact that protein is a "flexible macronutrient" — that is, it can be converted into calories or muscle — is the reason why it's important to keep protein intake high when you're in a calorie deficit. If your body thinks it can break your muscle down into protein, and then convert that protein into calories, it will. So keep the weight-lifting intense, and the protein consumption high.

Why a Calorie Deficit is Necessary

Back to the question. Your total body fat content can be expressed as a caloric number. For example, if you have 40 pounds of body fat, and a pound of body fat contains 3,500 calories, then you have 140,000 calories of body fat. Nobody can lose all their fat (nor should they).

We have fat in our brains and in our internal organs that is necessary for bodily function. So even the most shredded people you see probably have 8-10 pound of "unseen" body fat.

So, let's say you want to lose 30 pounds of body fat. At the end of that loss, you'd be ready for a Muscle & Fitness magazine cover shoot.

To lose 30 pounds, you have to accomplish a 105,000 calorie deficit. That might sound like a lot, but it's not. If you accomplish a 700-800 calorie deficit every day, you could accomplish that deficit easily in 4 months.

Combined with the water weight you'd lose, you'd probably be down 40 pounds in that time. The goal of the daily calorie deficit is really to hit a much bigger calorie deficit over a longer period of time, breaking it up into daily chunks.

Think of your body like a stock market, opening when you wake up and closing when you go to sleep. Your body settles accounts at the end of the day. Remember the two basic ways to achieve a calorie deficit:

> (1)Move more.
> (2)Eat less.

It doesn't matter how much of it was from fat, or how much of it was from carbs. Your fat stores don't care if you ate 38 stalks of broccoli or drank 5 small Shamrock Shakes (both 1900 calories).

The only thing that matters for fat loss is: did you expend more calories than you consumed? If so, your body will take it out of your fat. If not, you won't lose fat. It's that simple.

13

If I eat too little, won't my body go into "starvation mode"?

I don't know what "starvation mode" is. But if I had to guess, it's something fitness bloggers have invented to keep you returning to their diets (kind of like gyms that have "pizza day" on Fridays) — it makes the fat loss process sound more complicated than it is.

You're not a PC computer — you don't have a "starvation mode." If you are in a calorie deficit while maintaining your muscle mass, you will lose fat.

If you're not losing fat, it's because you're either eating too much or moving too little. Not if you're eating a pound of protein per pound of bodyweight while lifting weights.

It's very important that you don't think your fitness knowledge will somehow bend the laws of physics. Fat is stored energy. No amount of "fitness hacks" besides creating an energy imbalance (expending more calories than you consume) will result in fat loss.

14

How do I calculate how many calories I'm consuming?

Again, use one of two apps — either MyFitnessPal or MyPlate. They have foods pre-logged in the app. And you can also enter custom foods.

Track everything. If you track everything except for your mayonnaise and late night peanut butter snack, you could "track" a 500 calorie deficit, but in reality you're in a 100 calorie surplus.

That's why it's so important to round up when it comes to food and round down when it comes to your TDEE and calorie deficit.

The more "room" you give yourself in your calculations, the better chance you have of fooling yourself you're in a calorie deficit when you're really not.

Fast-forward 12 weeks, and all you've done is spend hundreds of hours counting calories and lifting weights to no end (as many do their entire lives).

15

Is it okay to try "intuitive eating" instead of calorie counting?

Yes! You are free to train as you wish. But my "intuition" is that a 20% caloric surplus won't be "intuitive."

Eating less is very hard. It's not going to feel good. You're not going to like it. Fat loss won't feel "natural." A cut is not "intuitive."

Your body will be fighting you the entire 12 weeks. Your body wants to reach homeostasis. It doesn't want to lose fat. It wants to be comfortable. It wants to escape the stress of caloric restriction.

For the time of your cut, if your goal is maximum fat loss while retaining maximum health, it's going to be a fight to the death in your soul between your intuition and your discipline to meet your goals.

Try "intuitive eating" when you've maintained your goal body fat percentage. Not during a cut. Don't experiment with diets, have them fail to supply fat loss, and then write off dieting together.

The path I'm giving you is a smart and healthy way. Either commit to it, or don't — but don't modify key principles and then bemoan the lack of results. Deficit. Lifting. Protein.

Part 3

CAR

DIO

16

How much cardio do I have to do in order to get in shape?

1. Cardio Isn't Necessary, But It Really Helps

First of all, cardio isn't necessary, but it makes hitting a calorie deficit a lot easier. It's easier to get the picture with a graph, as usual.

Remember: Your BMR (Basal Metabolic Rate) is what your particular body burns throughout the day just maintaining itself (what it would burn in a coma).

Your TDEE is your BMR calories plus the calories from all your activity — chewing calories burned, breathing calories burned, cardio calories burned, every calorie burned on top of your basic calories.

Let's take my body as an example — I'm a 200 pound, 6 foot, 29 year old male. Add up all my weight lifting together, and I lift weights for about 5 hours per week. Add up all my cardio (fast walking or running), and I do about 1.5 hours of cardio per week. Here are what my calories look like visually:

BMR =2000
TDEE =2700
TDEE + Cardio =3000

Cardio and Calories-Burned

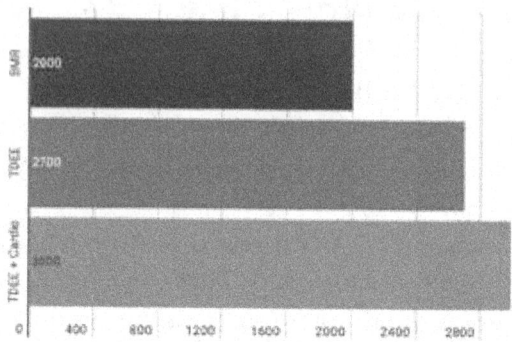

How does Cardio help with a deficit? Well, if I took a 24-hour nap and took only a short break to eat 2500 calories per day, I would be in a 500-calorie surplus.

But if we were active all day and lifted weights, and still consumed 2500 calories, I would be in a 200 calorie deficit. At that rate, I would lose 1400 calories per week.

And since a pound of fat is 3500 calories, it would take me a little under 3 weeks to lose a pound of fat. And that's with lifting weights.

But if I do cardio every day — let's say I burn 300 calories during a cardio session — then I'm in a 500 calorie deficit! If this is all confusing, look at this chart:

Cardio and Calorie Deficit

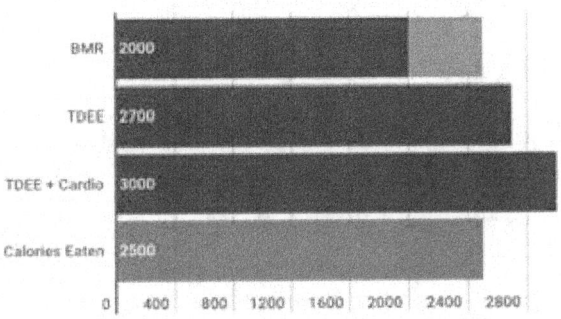

Notice that cardio pushes my calorie deficit 500 calories past my "Calories Eaten." At this rate, I will lose a pound per week if I do a 300-calorie cardio session each day.

at means cardio can triple your rate of fat loss, simply by burning 300 extra calories per day. To put this into perspective, if I were to run a marathon, I would burn 3,500 calories.

But I probably wouldn't be able to run for a week. Doing smaller cardio sessions that don't require as much recovery can be as effective as running one marathon per week.

Do you know what else is 3,500 calories? My favorite late-night college grab from McDonald's:

- Double Quarter Pounder
- Large Fries
- Large Coke
- 20 Piece McNuggets
- Apple Pie

No joke, I could consume that in the time it takes to watch the opening credits of Pineapple Express, which I often did. at's a marathon's worth of food.

You might not consume that much in one sitting, but how about in one day? How easy is it to eat 3500 calories? Very easy.

On your days when you do hit your diet on point, cardio can be the long-term habit that makes the big difference between starving yourself for a year (probably giving up before then), or seeing your abs in 12 weeks. Eating less is always easier than moving more (remember — some McDonald's meals can equal a marathon's worth of calories, especially if you are closer to 160 pounds).

But on the positive side, when you are hitting your deficit consistently, cardio can triple the speed that you see results.

2. Cardio "Calorie Calculators" Are Usually Wrong

We have to make a distinction between "net calories burned" and "gross calories burned." at is, if I took a nap for 30 minutes, I would burn about 40 calories in that 30 minute period.

Or, if I was up and active, hanging out with friends, I might be burning 80 calories during that 30 minutes. If I run for a half-hour at a 10-minute-mile pace, some "calorie calculators" will say I burned 400 calories on that 30-minute run.

But if I would have been burning 80 calories going about my daily routing during that half-hour regardless, then I really only burned an extra 320 calories. It's important to remember this.

3. Do the Cardio at Will Get Done

Do whatever cardio feels most comfortable to you. Don't worry about debates over high intensity and low intensity cardio. Track your calories — the cardio you can do every day is better than the cardio that you hate so much you stop after 2 days.

For example, I used to be really inconsistent with my cardio for one simple reason: I hated it. But the only cardio I felt comfortable doing was running. And in order to run, I'd have to blast heavy metal music.

And that was emotionally exhausting. And all for what? A few hundred calories? So I was in this habit of doing the most grueling exercise just for a few extra calories burned.

Then someone asked me, "Why don't you try briskly walking on a treadmill with a 5% incline?" Turns out, I could break a sweat on a 30 minute treadmill walk, and I'd burn the same calories as if I went on a 15 minute run. e only differences were:

(1) I wasn't mentally exhausted after the cardio, and (2) I was more consistent doing the cardio.

4. Always Do Cardio After Lifting Weights

If you're going to do cardio, never do it before you lift. This will make you weaker during your lifting session, and the whole point is to maintain strength and muscle. Always do cardio after weights.

The only exception to this is if you're going to lift in the afternoon, and you only have time to do cardio in the morning, that's fine. It shouldn't upset your weight routine that much.

17

Is it okay to do cardio instead of weight training?

Sure. You can do anything you want! But I have no idea what kind of fat loss results that will give you. My guess is you will end up a smaller version of your current self, with the same body fat percentage, and less muscle.

The Only Time It's Okay

Th only circumstance I would recommend doing cardio without weight lifting is if you register as "obese" and have a big learning curve. Focus on creating a calorie deficit first. is is 90% of the battle anyway.

And you probably already have a decent amount of lower body muscle. Shoot for an hour a day of something hard, even if that's an hour-long walk at a pace that gets your heart beating. Then try running for 5 minutes, walking for 15. en try running for 5, walking for 10.

Then try running for 10, walking for 10. Until you can run straight for 20 minutes. Once you can do that, start adding a weight routine as you are able.

When It's Not Okay

If you're just overweight, or have less than 60

pounds to lose, then you are in the zone to start doing weights and cardio.

Again, the reason for this is that we are not aiming to create a lifestyle in this cut. The goal is not to become a great swimmer, or a fast runner. The goal is to lose as much fat as possible in 12 weeks.

Don't focus on performance. Focus on maintaining your muscle so that your calorie deficit eats away at your fat tissues, rather than your muscle tissues (resulting in a skinny-fat you, rather than a shredded you).

18

For cardio, should I sprint or walk?

This is an age-old debate. People will tell you:

"If you want to burn fat, you have to enter the fat-burning zone!!!!"

They will tell you that High Intensity Interval Training (HIIT), which is basically short bursts of sprints, is better than Low Intensity Steady State (LISS), like brisk walking and using the elliptical at a low resistance.

They will tell you that HIIT gives you an "afterburn" and you need to "optimize your cardio" by doing short springs instead of long walks.

Guess what? The fat-burning zone is about as real as the Phantom zone. There is not such thing as a fat- burning zone. The only reason to do cardio during a cut is to raise your TDEE a few hundred calories.

You're not trying to become an ultra-marathoner just yet. Leave performance goals to your six-pack self. Get the six-pack first, then you can focus on building endurance if that's something you want.

There is only one thing that burns fat. You know what it is. I've hammered it into you so far. A calorie deficit.

The Most Important Lesson From Cardio

ere is a really important lesson to be learned here. is lesson could be the difference between another failed diet and the shredded body you never thought you could have:

> Don't let the "perfect" become
> the enemy of the real.

Don't let someone's blog on "optimal fat-burning cardio" make you feel like you're wasting your time on the treadmill unless you're doing 30 minutes of sprints. Find something you like, and do that until it gets really hard. And then keep going.

I started doing 25 minutes on the treadmill after my weight session at 5% incline, at 4.0 miles per hour. Eventually, I alternated between 5 minutes at 5% incline and 5 minutes at 10% incline for 25 minutes.

Eventually, I made my way to 10% incline for 25 minutes, ending with 5 minutes at 11%. Find ways to turn something you like into a fat-melting workout.

But if it ever gets unbearable to the point where you start getting tempted to avoid cardio altogether, back off a little bit. Take the resistance down.

Do 5 or 10 minutes less. 200 calories burned every day for the next 12 weeks (16,800 calories — 5 extra pounds of fat) is better than one 500-calorie session done once a week (6,000 calories ... a little over a pound).

Don't let the idea of doing the best cardio get in the way of a sustainable habit. Do it. It could 3x the rate that you burn fat, and therefore 3x the amount of fat you lose over the same 12 week period.

19

An easy wat to 2x your cardio calories

Let's say you're doing 30 minutes of steady jogging every day after your lift weights, but you aren't losing fat fast enough.

For example, you might be a week into your cut with no weight loss to show for it. What's the deal? Most likely, you're either under-estimating the calories you're eating, or over-estimating your TDEE.

If you feel like you really can't eat any less, and you really can't work out any longer, here's a simple way to double the calories you burn during cardio: Tabata.

Tabata is when you devote 4 minutes to high-intensity bursts of cardio, with 20 seconds giving 100% intensity, and 10 seconds of rest. Over 4 minutes, you endure eight 20-second bursts of exercise. So, it looks like this: So, does one 4:00 Tabata set burn 2x the calories of a 30-minute jogging session? Unfortunately, no. But 4 minutes of Tabata burns way more calories than 4 minutes of low-intensity cardio.

Tabata Timetable	
0:00	Burst #1
0:20	10-second rest
0:30	Burst #2
0:50	10-second rest
1:00	Burst #3
1:20	10-second rest
1:30	Burst #4
1:50	10-second rest
2:00	Burst sprint #5
2:20	10-second rest
2:30	Burst #6
2:50	10-second rest
3:00	Burst #7
3:20	10-second rest
3:30	Burst #8

Takeaway:

Substitute 12 minutes of jogging for 3 sets of Tabata, and then do 20 minutes of jogging (or some other form of low-intensity cardio, like elliptical).

So, your cardio would look like this:

Modified Cardio	
Tabata #1	4 Minutes
Tabata #2	4 Minutes
Tabata #3	4 Minutes
Low-Intensity Cardio	20 minutes

Here are a list of Tabata exercises you can do that will help you to shed fat even faster. Remember, it's 20- seconds on, 10-seconds off, repeated 8 times.

- Easier
    - Plank
    - Rowing Machine
    - Captain'sChairLegRaises
- Harder
    - Burpees
    - High-KneeStationarySprints
    - Push-Ups
    - HangingLeg-Raises

Part 4

DISC IPL INE

20

What kind of emotional roller coaster should I expect during a cut?

Not gonna lie — it gets pretty bad. Your brain runs on glucose and ketones. There are certain non-essential parts of the brain that your body will start to neglect. One of them is your limbic system — it's basically the part of your brain that regulates your mood.

is is the perspective you need to keep: When your mood starts to crash because of hunger, that's when your body is beginning to use its own fat as fuel for energy. Don't get duped by your hunger into eating so that you can feel better. Nutritionists will say:

"Your brain runs on energy! It's unhealthy to cut calories, because your body needs energy to be healthy!"

When you hear your "Inner Nutritionist" telling you to give yourself calories so that you can be "healthy," I want you to do something. Look at your belly button. Do it right now. Grab the fat right under your belly button, with your thumb and your pointer finger. Jiggle it.

THAT'S YOUR ENERGY!

You don't need food to energize your body. The whole point of a cut is that you have excess energy inside your body that you're trying to get rid of.

You will often be tempted to eat so that you can fix your mood. Don't do it. Let your body fix your own mood. Saying "No" to food is hard. It's hard on your body. You're going to be stressed.

People will tell you "It's time for a Snickers." Mood crashing is just part of being energy deprived. It's part of having a starving limbic system. It's a way of your weak brain crying out for help.

But guess what — you're not starving. Your body is just throwing a temper tantrum. You need to learn to say "No" to yourself. This is very hard. Life becomes harder when your body is pulling calories from your belly, love handles, thighs, and neck to keep you going.

Find other ways to boost your mood. Find zero- calorie snacks that you can enjoy. Amp up on caffeine. Or maybe do the opposite, and drink some Slenderizer tea, or some oolong tea. Meditate. Go for a walk.

Just don't let your mood talk you into breaking your deficit. An idle mind is a moody mind. Go find a way to work or relax that operationalizes your energy.

However, if you are having major mood swings

because of your calorie deficit, you may be eating in a way that isn't optimal for your body. For example, you may need to eat 5 meals a day, rather than 1 big meal a day, if it helps your mood remain normal throughout the day.

21

How do I recover after I've blown my calorie deficit with a food binge?

This is really tough. You'll want to hate yourself. To blame yourself. To punish yourself. Don't. We tend to think that if we aren't very harsh with ourselves, then we would indulge all the time.

But that's not the case.

One study showed that among students who procrastinated for an exam in class, those who punished themselves were more likely to procrastinate for the next exam! e students who practiced self-compassion were more likely to prepare ahead of time for the next exam.

Think about it this way. You doing this cut is supposed to be an act of self-love. You're trying to better yourself. You're trying to do something good for yourself, because you are worthy of being invested in, of being made healthy. You are worthy of a better body.

The idea of "punishing" yourself will create a sense of self-hatred that will actually push you to indulge in high-calorie food so that you can soothe the negative emotion. So a binge creates another binge. And then you're on the brink of giving up altogether.

Don't punish yourself. In fact, I'll go this far: Make a night of it.

Remember this:

Failure is never a good reason to abandon your fitness goals.

Failure is just a reminder why you made the goals.

One day, I was hovering around 1500 calories at 4:00pm, and I hadn't eaten dinner yet. My calorie goal was 2,000 calories. After a hard workout and a grueling cardio session, I was starving.

So I binged. What was my weakness?

Oh, nothing that bad. Just a bowl of Cheerios and some skim milk. A healthy snack, right?

2 cups of cheerios plus a cup of skim milk is 190 calories. Okay, up to 1790. How would I fit dinner into 210 calories? I started panicking. I started hating myself for eating the bowl of Cheerios. So, what did I do?

Poured another huge-ass bowl of cheerios without even thinking. I didn't think "Screw it!" I just thought, "Oh it's only one more. And I did work out so hard today." 210 more calories.

And then ... like I was a zombie walking into a nursery, I just started eating. And eating. And eating. Five bowls later (seven total) ... I'm at 3000 calories. UGH.

I felt like crap about myself. So I went for a run, and I threw up. And then I ordered a large pizza, sat on the couch, and ate the whole thing while watching Jessica Jones on Netflix.

I felt numb. But beneath the numb, I felt like a weak, pathetic loser. But I've learned a better way to deal with things. We can't let ourselves go down the road of self-punishment. at will never get us in shape.

That same situation happened again about a week later, except this time it was with a pizza a family member had left in the house, left over from a part. Only about 30 minutes old. Smelled amazing.

I could indulge, going way over my calorie limit. And I realized, I had a choice: I can indulge in this thing and completely hate myself. Or, I can enjoy the hell out of it.

So, I set my table. Opened up Netflix. Made a salad to go with it. Opened a Stella Artois. Opened the box. Pressed play. And delighted in that pizza. It was so much more satisfying. No guilt. Because before I indulged, I decided to enjoy it.

Now I have a rule for myself. In the future, if I get the sense that I'm going to binge, and I really have no say in the matter (and there are those nights), make a night of it. My rule is basically:

No guilty binges.

Now, you might be thinking, "If I have that perspective, I'll binge all the time!" No. Remember: you love yourself. Binging all the time isn't a good way to love yourself.

Investing your health is a good way to love yourself. But in those crazy, out-of-control, this-is-really- happening moments, force yourself to take it slow, and to enjoy it.

Chances are, by enjoying it fully — by letting yourself melt into your enjoyment of the food — you likely may not even eat as much as if you were scarfing it down like a jackal (like I did with Cheerios).

Don't see it as "Oh what the hell, I might as well eat this pizza because I'm a big fat fatty." No. If you want to, you should eat the rest of the pizza. But do it out of self- love. ENJOY IT!

Love yourself.

And then get back to investing in your health, with fond memories of your enjoyment of food, and a renewed dedication to your 12- week cut, knowing your standards are only very rigid for a little while.

And, if it helps, walk at 4.0 on an incline on your treadmill for a full hour tomorrow after your weights. Nothing heavy. No crazy commitments. Just something to balance out the damage. It will be your on-ramp back into health, into a deficit, into your cut.

The most important thing to remember is this: Failure is not a good reason to abandon your fitness goals. One failure — heck, a thousand failures — is not a sufficient reason to give up!

But I want you to remember something else. Let's say you're about to binge. Let's say you already bought the pizza. You already paid for the ice cream cone. You already drove to the restaurant. You already opened the bottle of beer.

You have to remember: *You don't have to consume it!* You haven't eaten it yet! I remember I once bought an ice cream cone while I was trying to hit my calorie deficit.

I was doing well for the day, but the ice cream would have busted my deficit. I got a medium. I put chocolate sprinkles on it. I even took the first bite. It was so good.

But I had a moment of clarity:
> *"I don't have to finish this."*

So I took one more bite. And then I took my finger and swiped the entire ice cream portion of my treat into the garden, leaving a cone with some ice cream inside of it. I ate that. 200 calories vs. the 800 I would have consumed. I went for a 2 mile walk. The 25% deficit was saved.

Remember: you don't have to finish something just

because you bought it. You don't have to buy the Wendy's nuggets just because they're 99 cents.

Most foods that you can buy for cheap come at the highest caloric cost. Don't eat it. Throw it away.

Put one slice on a plate, and put the rest in the freezer. Get out of the mindset that you have to "clear your plate" by shoving it down your gullet. You don't. is is the hardest moment to remember your fitness goal, but it is the most important one.

22

How do I motivate myself to go to the gym?

This is a really important question. At the end of the day, you could be the Einstein of fitness, but all that knowledge wouldn't help you if you never did the work. But that's the hard part.

> Showing up to the gym.
> Putting down the ice cream cone.
> Getting the workout in.

Here are a few tips to help you actually make it to the gym:

1. Forget "Motivation"

We've all Googled "How to get motivated to go to the gym," right? Well, that's the least effective method of actually getting to the gym. ink about it. You want your gym-activities to be consistent, right?

Well, what's more inconsistent than motivation? Your strategy for consistency can't be "Bring my level of motivation to a level of consistency that matches my goals." No. You'll never be as motivated as your goals need you to be.

Essentially: your discipline can't be about your motivation. It has to be about discipline.

The shortest, straightest line to your goal body is finishing the next rep, the next mile, the next deficit.

Motivations change. If you only worked out when you had the motivation, you'd work out every January 1st, and the occasional May 1st when you realize summer is immanent.

You don't need motivation. You need discipline. You need the ability to go to the gym when you have no motivation. And guess what: There is no shortcut to saying "no" to yourself. ere is no lifehack to discipline.

It's like a muscle. It grows or it atrophies. You do the thing, or you don't do the thing. ere is no existential soul searching that will automatically give you more willpower, any more than it will give you bigger muscles. It won't. Do the work.

There is not shortcut. And the biggest roadblock to discipline is thinking there are shortcuts, and trying to figure them out. ere aren't. Bulldoze through your emotions. Clobber your excuses.

The shortest, straightest line to your fitness goal is doing the next rep, running the next mile, hitting the next calorie deficit.

2. Use a Pre-Workout

A Pre-Workout is a supplement you can take that is half- Monster energy drink, half-scientifically proven performance enhancing substances. Nothing illegal. Nothing harmful. Just your usual suspects — caffeine, taurine, arginine, Beta-Alanine, etc. My favorite two Pre- Workout supplements are called "N.O. Xplode" (by B.S.N.) and "Pulse" (by Legion Athletics).

If you take 1 or 2 scoops of this, mixed with 8 oz. of water, you will go to the gym. Not because it motivates you. But because you start to feel your skin tingling. You start to feel your blood rushing. Your brain has an exhilarating surge of focus. It's a powerful neuroenhancer.

But more importantly: if you take a Pre-Workout

and don't workout, you will feel like absolute crap. You won't be able to sleep. You won't be able to relax.

Your body will be so full of energy, you will be compelled to release it through exercise. And there's nothing more fun than working out on 2 scoops of N.O. Xplode.

3. Start a 30-Day Program

Sometimes, we are unmotivated to go to the gym because we're really not sure what to do there. We go, we fool around, we throw some weights around, we hit the treadmill for a mile or so, and we walk out.

But what if you could find a way of working out that left you shaking and exhausted after every workout? The best way to do that is to go to bodybuilding.com, and search their programs — my personal favorite right now is Craig Capurso's "30 Days Out," where he has a video each day for 30 days that you follow.

It's for all fitness levels, and he shows you exactly what to do for every single second of a one-hour workout for 30 days straight.

Finding a workout program on bodybuilding.
com will give you the structure you need to follow.
No leaving the gym early. No dreading the gym
because you don't know what to do.

You go to the gym, and you do what the guy says
to do in the video, and you go home. No more.
No less. Your goal at the gym then isn't to "get in
shape," but to complete the prescribed workout. A
lot less pressure, a lot more sustainable, and over
the long hall, a lot better results.

4. Find Something You Like

I'm good at two things when it comes to fitness:
Pressing and Ditance Running. This means that,
for my weight, I can "push" a lot of weight on the
bench press compared to most average people who
weigh 200 pounds.

I can also run 5 miles at a 9 minute pace
with moderate ease. Neither of these feats is
extraordinary. I know a lot of people who can push
more than me and run faster than me.

But because I feel strong when I do them, I can
tolerate doing them each day. at's what I try to do
when I go to the gym each day — find one workout
that I'm really good at, and start the day with

that. It gets me into the groove of the workout, and I push it hard, lots of reps, and show off my performance.

Then, I hit all the other exercises I need to do for the day, knowing that they will help me get stronger on my favorite exercise.

Find something you like to do, make it the cornerstone of your routine, and give yourself something to look forward to at the gym.

23

Can you give me a less time-consuming workout?

The dangerous thing about "minimizing" workouts is that it can reinforce a sedentary lifestyle — most of us do have to sit down all day to do non-active things, like paperwork, reading, and writing. But if there's a week or two in your life when you *simply don't have time to exercise,* then yes. It's called a "7 Minute Workout."

Let's say you're busy for a week and won't have any time to go to the gym. Commit to doing two 7 minute workouts per day. You can Google them, and there are many "7 Minute Workout" apps you can use.

But the principle is that, unlike the gym, in which you lift weights, take a break, lift weights, take a break, lift weights, take a break, etc. — there is no break in a 7 Minute Workout. It's a full-body workout. And here's a sample, published in *The New York Times:*

1. Jumping Jacks   20
2. Wall Sit   20 seconds
3. Push-Up   20
4. Abdominal Crunch   20
5. Step-up onto chair   20 (each leg)
6. Squat   20
7. Triceps dip on-chair   20
8. Plank   20 seconds
9. High knees running in place   20 seconds
10. Lunge   20 (each leg)
11. Push-up   20
12. Side plank   20 seconds (each side)

Start a timer right before you begin your jumping jacks. If you take less than 7 minutes to complete this 12-part exercise sequence, simply repeat the sequence. If you are extremely fit, simply aim to complete this sequence as many times as possible within 7 minutes.

24
Why do I keep breaking my diet?

There is only one answer: You make excuses. What is the magic bullet for strictly adhering to your diet? What is the simple path to consistent fat loss? What is the only way to get shredded? ere's only one answer. It's not a product. It's not a specific diet ratio. It's not a "life hack." It's not a program. It's very simple:

Stop making excuses.

ere is no cheat code. Eating less (and moving more) is a primal test of your willpower. We are tempted to eat calorie-dense foods (foods that are high-calorie, but don't make us feel full), and then complain about how little food we're allowed to eat. In order to use willpower, you have to understand that willpower is a muscle, and you never face any dietary situations that are "too heavy" for your willpower muscle.

However, if you want to make dietary adherence easier, there are a couple secrets that food marketers use to get you to break your diet — knowing them helps you to get out of the headlock they can put you in by tempting your cravings.

The Halo Effect

The first marketing trick is called "The Halo Effect," and it happens, for example, in the grocery store when the nice lady in the visor hands you a pig-in-a-blanket on a toothpick. "Why not?" So you indulge.

 Then, you go fill your basket with Romaine lettuce and chicken, and on your way back, you eat one more. "It's only one!" at's the halo effect: it shrouds dietary sinfulness in a veil of holiness. "Just one" is like sinking a fishhook into your appetite — "Just one" always translates into "one more."

What is the slogan of Lay's potato chips? "Bet you can't eat just one." So don't even start. Don't go down that road. Set the structure of your diet, and do not indulge in the "Just one" fallacy.

You're setting yourself up for defeat. What you justify as a "100 calorie indulgence" will translate into a 500 calorie compromise somewhere else. 12 mini-muffins don't equal 1 big muffin. They equal 4 big muffins.

Don't kid yourself. Put the "sample" down. Don't even reach for a "taste." Tasting always turns into

> *Don't "Just one" yourself. Hold strong. Be faithful to your aim.*
>
> *You know "Just one" is a lie that will make you feel terrible. It always is.*

gobbling. Stop. Don't. Look your friends dead in the eye and tell them: "I'm on a diet." Who cares what they think? They aren't the ones who made the commitment. You are. So order a water, eat your salad, and never tell yourself: "I deserve a taste."

The What-The-Hell Effect

The second marketing trick is called "The What-

The-Hell Effect," which is what happens after "The Halo Effect."

This psychological experience is what happens when you've allowed your diet to crack just a little bit. And that crack turns into a breach. It happened to me once at Applebee's. I was out with friends, they ordered mozzarella sticks.

You're not going to eat a mozzarella stick, I told myself. But I decide to Google in my phone: "Applebee's Mozzarella Stick Calories." 1 Serving: 900 calories. Yikes! ... Wait a second ... I adjusted the portion size to "1 Mozzarella Stick."

100 CALORIES! Yes!!!

I reached out, and took that first bite: the delicious cheese melted in my mouth, the crispy fried breading perfectly complementing it, coated with a zesty marinara dip that created an orgasmic flavor experience.

It was shamefully blissful.

Well ... damn. at was too good to have just one. at was amazing. What's the purpose of life anyway? Aren't we meant to enjoy things? Aren't we meant to be happy?

One mozzerella stick turned into a bacon cheeseburger and cheesecake.

Aren't we meant to savor the fruits of the earth? If I'm always "restricting" myself just to get in shape, I'll spend my whole life trying to become happy through fitness, but I'll never enjoy life. I need to relax a little bit. It's just one more stick. 100 calories here, 100 calories there. What's the big deal?

I opened my menu, flipped to the burger section, and ordered my forbidden fruit:

Triple Bacon Burger with a loaded baked potato and a Blue Moon ... with a slice of cheesecake to finish. Not counting the mozzarella sticks, it was 2700 calories. I ate my TDEE for dinner.

But it started with one mozzarella stick. Just one. "What the hell! ... Garf-Snarb-Blarg." Don't "Just one more" yourself, because if you do, you'll probably "What the hell" your diet — a one-way ticket to regret, self-loathing, and further reinforcing the idea that you could never really get in shape.

You can get in shape. You must. The longer you keep your diet, the easier it gets. Dieting is not an uphill battle that gets harder every day. The longer you go, the better you get at it. If you mess up a few times, the best thing you can do is not to beat yourself up, but to start over immediately.

The reason you keep breaking your diet is because you keep making excuses to say "One more." Nobody ever decides, while they're doing well on their diet, "I'm going to break my diet and eat 3,000 calories in one sitting!"

They're dragged there blindly and violently by their desires. Don't be dragged there. Don't bite the hook of "I deserve this." It will be serving you up for dinner.

Part 5

DIET

25
Isn't it better to eat 5 times a day to "keep your metabolsim going?"

No. It doesn't matter how many "meals" you eat per day. e only thing that matters is the amount of calories you consume. Temet nosce — Know thyself, like the oracle tells Neo in the Matrix. Do you function better with 5 meals per day? Eat 5 meals per day. Do you function better eating only one big meal at the end of the day (like me)? en do that. Experiment.

This is a good point to call out all of the "authoritative" fitness blogs that say you have to keep eating throughout the day to "keep your metabolic engine running."

Dude. You're fat. You have the fuel. You don't need to "carb up" or any stupid crap like that.

Every fitness guru on the internet is going to try to sell you their "best way" to get in shape — the optimal path to your ultimate physique. It's all

B.S.

The only factor for fat loss is caloric deficit. You might be able to "hack" a few calories off your total TDEE by eating meals at the right times, or separating meals into different food groups, but those are pennies-on-the-dollar compared to the fat-loss value of eating less than you burn.

So, in summary, eat the number of meals that makes it easiest for you to hit your calorie deficit for the day.

That's the only rule. Don't let anyone tell you that you "have to" eat carbs at a certain hour, or never eat carbs and fat together, or eat 5 meals a day to keep the engine running. ey're hokey ways for so-called fitness professionals to sell pseudo-knowledge.

There's a 20 billion dollar industry devoted to coming up with empty nuance and selling it (ever read the magazine Men's Fitness? It's all crap).

You don't need to follow the same principles an NFL football player follows. He burns 10,000 calories a day. He gets to eat differently. If you want to look like you play in the NFL, you're better off eating like a ballerina for a short period of time than a football player.

"Eat big to get big" is a middle-school slogan that never got anyone looking shredded. It's not popular, but it's what you need to do: "Eat small to look big." Trust me. e path to more is less. And thank God, the principles behind fat loss are simple:

Hit your calorie deficit.

"Just one" always turns into "just one more."

Don't worry about anything else. Don't buy anyone's program, or get click-baited into "the one meal-timing rule that's keeping you fat." Hit your deficit. Everything else is a sales ploy.

26

How do I practically hit my protein goal?

If you're struggling to hit your protein goal, there are a few things you can do.

First, purchase a protein supplement. This could be a powder that you mix, or a pre-made drink. Whatever you do, make sure that there are not more than 2-3g of carbs and fat in the formula. If you're struggling to hit your deficit and your protein goal at the same time, you want your protein to be as lean as possible.

Second, batch cook chicken and eat one breast per day. This won't be sufficient to hit your goal, but it will make hitting your goal with "regular" food much easier, knowing you have a 40-50g bump coming later in the day.

Third, examine your protein sources—ensure that they are not fatty, carby lures in disguise. A lot of people think that if there is a protein-sounding word in the food's name, then the food is all protein. This is false.

For example, I used to think that General Tso's chicken was a good source of protein — because, you know, *it's chicken*. I was a deeply confused man. General Tso's chicken is about 10% protein, and mostly fat and carbs. So, ensure your current "sources" of protein are lean, meaning they are mostly composed of protein.

27

Are there any supplements that are helpful during the cut?

There's a very good website called *MuscleForLife.com* that gives detailed explanations of helpful supplements for weight loss.

I trust this website, because they are committed to highlighting fraud in the supplement community, and are extremely transparent about their sources and manufacturing for the supplements that they sell.

In other words, this site is devoted to educating you about supplements (their supplement line is called "Legion"), and they leave it up to you to find other supplements if they better fit your liking.

I recommend reading the research on that website. If you're looking for fat loss help, I recommend their supplements Pheonix and Forge.

However, the cornerstone of a cut will have a good whey protein — Legion's Whey+ or IsoPure are good whey protein brands. e brand doesn't matter so much, as long as it is low-carb and low-fat (to keep the calories down).

If you don't have a whey protein powder mix, it's very hard to hit your protein goal. And if you don't hit your protein goal while in a 25% calorie deficit, you risk your body converting your muscle into energy, which is the opposite of what we want (remember, we don't want "weight loss" — we want fat loss; this makes us different from the anorexics).

So — buy a whey protein shake. Other than that, be careful when buying "fat burning" pills. There are very bad companies out there that sell unhealthy pills, but Legion sells good supplements that are healthy and really do aid in fat loss.

28
How do I prepare my meals to save time?

The best way to prepare your meals, especially if you are short on time, is to buy 7-days worth of Tupperware, and cook everything in one night. Utilize your oven, or grill if you have one. ese are the two best appliances for "mass cooking." For example, you could buy these four products that could last you the entire week:

- 10 Pounds of Chicken ($50)
- 5 One-Bags of Frozen Broccoli ($15)
- 4 Four-Packs of Triple-Zero Yogurt ($15)
- 4 Four-Packs of Sugar-Free Jello ($15)
- 3 16-oz. Spring Mix Containers ($20)
- Fat-free dressing ($3)
- 3-Pound Whey Protein Powder ($30)
- 36-Pack Water Bottles ($10)

Roast in your oven all the chieken and broccoli, portion it, and here's what you'll have for each day:

- 1.3 Pounds of chicken
- Half-Pound of Broccoli
- 2 Triple-Zero Yogurts
- 2 Sugar-Free Jello Packs
- A large, 8-oz. salad.
- 2 Whey Protein Shakes
- 5 Water Bottles

By the way, this entire week's worth of food costs

$160, averaging $22 per day. If you were to buy these meals at a "health meal" store, you'd be paying $50 per day.

But here, all it takes is an oven and a timer. There's really no excuse not to eat foods that are healthy and conducive to a calorie deficit, especially when they're affordable and easy to prepare a week's-worth in a single night.

29
What if someone wants to cook me a meal?

Easy. I know it's embarrassing to count calories. People usually think it's weird. So if you don't feel comfortable asking your host what the calories are in the meal they make, make that meal your only meal of the day and exercise discernment when you eat.

Try to guess what each food is, log it, and enter it in your app.

If you walk away feeling you met your calorie deficit, great. If not, cut a few hundred calories from your deficit the next few days.

Track calories afterward in your app of choice. It's okay to eat someone else's cooking. But don't let it serve as an excuse to "blow your diet" for a night. No. *The diet is still on.*

If they keep pushing 2nd helpings, 3rd helpings, 4th cake slices on you (hopefully you don't make it to your 3rd slice of cake), say "No thanks." One single, small helping of everything. at's it. It's simple. Not easy, but simple.

Dieters often feel that they are inconveniencing others with their embarrassing secret: "I'm on a diet." But people are very understanding. I find that, more often than not, people want to respect your diet, and often feel bad that they didn't know you were dieting if they just happen to find out later.

Hosts generally like to accommodate your guests. So, if they ask what kind of food your diet accommodates, just tell them: "It's pretty flexible, just lean meats and vegetables, and no processed sugar." That should limit their menu quite a bit, all the way from appetizers to dessert.

30
What if I have to eat at a restaurant?

Same as above. Make it your only meal. Stay away from sauces and gravies. Try to guess what you're eating and exercise discernment while consuming.

Track calories afterward in your app of choice. Don't let it become a norm. Restaurants are diet disasters waiting to happen — they are trying to make you buy more food.

They will make your hunger even worse. They smother everything in butter. Order a salad, no cheese, no croutons, dressing on the side.

Stay away from restaurants as much as possible for the entire duration of your cut.

31

How do I eat healthy while travelling?

This can be extremely hard. You are bombarded with marketing and smells from the tastiest, saltiest, sweetest, savoriest foods in the world. McDonald's. Sbarro — Ah, I love Sbarro!!!!!

Their pizza. Their calzones. Ugh, I just want to eat an entire meatball calzone with extra cheese.

Or heck, I'd take a hot slice of pepperoni with an ice-cold Diet Coke. Nothing is more tempting than eating fast food while travelling.

> At the airport.
> At the rest stops.

ou're basically a sitting duck for these companies' marketing teams. While you're waiting for your plane, or walking to the restroom, they pay millions of dollars to craft a smell or location so that you are assaulted with the constant voice in your head:

"Burger so yummy."
"Chicken so crispy."
"Cheese so gooey."
"Fries so crispy."

Don't do it!! You simply cannot eat healthy while travelling. I want you to follow one simple rule:

Do not buy anything.

Nothing. No bananas. No burgers. No beers. No nothing — er, anything. You can wait. It's that simple. You're not going to starve to death. You're just not. I promise. Are you travelling to a deserted island? Okay, if you're on a deserted island, barter for what food you need. But besides that, buy nothing.

Eat nothing. Be hungry. It's good for your mind. *It's good for your body.* And you'll work up a great calorie deficit. Take travel as an opportunity to practice restraint — like walking across coals. It is a feat that requires a lot of willpower.

Now, I already know you're reading this thinking, "You're ridiculous. I'm not putting myself through that. I'm not putting my family through that." Okay. Fair enough. Here are two things I'll let you buy (or bring with you) while traveling:

(1) Beef Jerky.
(2) Water.

That's it. Eat them. Enter your calories. You're good to go. Limit yourself to those two items. Don't eat the sample at the rest stop Starbucks. Don't eat the crackers they offer you on the plane.

Eat nothing. Be hungry. You won't die. It's actually good for you.

When the stewardess shoves those cookies in your face, you say: "NO THANK YOU!" Very rudely, like a celebrity might.

Okay, you don't have to be rude. But say it. Practice saying it in the mirror:

> "No thank you."
> "No thank you."
> "No cookies for me, thank you."
> "No crackers, thanks."
> "Just water."
> "No peanuts, just water, thanks."

You're not weak. You're strong. Give your six pack a chance.

You don't have to mean it. You just have to say it. You've got your beef jerky and your water. at is enough. at is all you need. Sound hard?

Losing fat is hard. But you can do this. You can do it. It is within your grasp. Beneath those flabs you can grab with your full fist is a six pack waiting to show itself to the world, waiting to meet the sun for the first time in decades, or ever.

Give your six pack a chance. Don't let travel convince you that you're weaker than you really are. You're not weak. You're strong. And there's a lean, muscular you waiting beneath your snowman figure, and he can't wait to meet the sun.

32
Should I eat more on days I train more?

No. Your TDEE is based on how many times you exercise per week. The fact that you take one or two days off from the gym is *already factored into your TDEE*. Eat the same calorie amount every day. As long as the information you entered into your TDEE calculator remains true, assume that it is indeed your TDEE.

If your calculator gave you a TDEE average of 2500, and you're aiming for a 20% deficit, eat no more than 2,000 calories, even if you "did extra work" at the gym.

> Stick to your number.
> Don't treat yourself.

You're only stealing time and work from your future self. Give your future self a gift by sticking to your calorie goal: *a head start on the body you've always wanted* ... instead of a roadblock.

33
What's a good 7-day meal plan?

Before we answer this question, you have to answer a question for yourself:

> Do you want to enjoy yourself as much as possible over the next 14 days, or do you want to lose as much fat as possible over the next 14 days?

If you're always trying to make yourself as comfortable as possible, always trying to have the finest experiences, always trying to get the tastiest experience of food, you'll never get in shape. Make the choice right now for the next 14 days: Fun, or fat loss?

> Don't B.S. yourself. Choose.

What's your goal? Is it to eat the tastiest food, or to make a real difference in your life and finally start getting in shape? Don't try to "have it all." Get in the mindset: Your goal is to get in shape. *Forget fun.* Forget flavor. Give it up.

This is the first rule of diet that will result in lasting fat loss:

> *Commit to boring.*

If you haven't put this book down yet, then I'll let you in on some ways you can still have tasty food while you diet. But your mantra for your cut is: Healthy, boring food. Healthy, boring food. Hit your calorie deficit. That's your goal. Don't focus your energy on constructing the "tastiest" diet possible. Focus on adherence, not exuberance.

The best way I've found to commit to a calorie deficit is to give yourself as little wiggle room as possible. is means that you need to choose one meal, and eat it every single day. That's your 7-day meal plan. A single meal that gets you to your calorie deficit x 7. That's it.

Here are a few options:

14-Day Option 1		
Chicken Breast	Dannon Triple-Zero Yogurt	BBQ Sauce
Roasted Broccoli	Sweet Potatoes	Apple
Spring Mix	Egg Whites	Halo Top Ice Cream
14-Day Option 2		
London Broil Steak	Siggi's Yogurt	A1 Steak Sauce
Zucchini	Toast	Orange
Romaine Lettuce	Turkey Bacon	Sugar-Free Jello
14-Day Option 3		
99% Lean Ground Turkey	Dannon Light and Fit Yogurt	Spaghetti Sauce
Brussels Sprouts	Pasta	Banana
Arugula Salad	Canadian Bacon	Sugar-Free Pudding

Remember: *how much* of these foods you eat is dependent on your activity level and weight. You must determine your TDEE and calculate your deficit goal, and determine how much of each food you need to eat.

But here's the trick. Commit to only eating the foods in your option-group. Maybe buy these foods at the grocery store, and only return to the grocery store in order to replenish these items specifically.

If you run into logistical issues with your family, and they don't want to eat the same thing every day, then you must explain to them that you've got special meals you eat for this time — is your health a priority or not?

If it helps, cook all 7 day's worth of food in a single sitting on Sunday night, and put it in Tupperware containers that you take with you to work or school throughout the week.

Leave as few opportunities to indulge up to your future self. Commit: I'm only eating these foods, and I'm hitting my calorie deficit by only eating these foods.

If you're the kind of person who can eat whatever they want — donuts, pizza, soda, McDonald's, etc. — and still have the self-control to hit your calorie deficit, more power to you! But I love to eat. I love to feel full.

The only thing that makes me feel full is eating a lot of food. at's why I eat low-calorie foods: so that I don't go to bed hungry at night. And committing myself to eating only these foods

keeps me from going over my budget.
Your best shot at getting in shape is to commit
to boring. One tip to spice things up: trade
your sauces for spices. All condiments, butter,
margarine, alfredo sauce, etc. — cut it out.

Instead, use spices like pepper, turmeric, oregano,
etc. They are zero-calorie ways to add flavor to
your food. So, while you're committed to boring,
you can find ways to add tolerable taste to your
food so that you go insane. But don't be in the
"maximize flavor" mindset — it will lead you into a
mindset of indulgence.

Commit to repetition.

Commit to boring.

34

How many carbs can I eat during a cut?

I just picture Dr. Evil right here — "… One *billion* carbs."

Okay, not a billion. at would be 4 billion calories, not counting the protein and fat you consumed along with the carbs. Even one thousand carbs would be 4,000 calories, which would take a 200-pound man to run a marathon in order to burn that amount.

At this point, it shouldn't surprise you to hear: It doesn't matter how many carbs you eat, as long as you're in a calorie deficit. However, there are a couple reasons to decrease your carbs.

1. Carbs are easy to eat.

Processed sugar especially — it's easy to eat muchos carbos without even thinking about it. Proof: all our favorite foods. Cup of ice-cream: 400 calories. McDonald's fries: 400 calories. Bowl of raisin bran with skim milk: 400 calories. You get it. Carbs are easy to eat without even noticing. So "cutting carbs" from out diet can help us to decrease our calories from our diet that we didn't even realize we were consuming.

2. Carbs are easily stored as fat.

Carbs, fat, and protein all have certain levels of energy efficiency.

Carbs are an extremely efficient form of energy — it takes little energy to digest complex carbs (like broccoli and sweet potatoes), and almost not energy to digest simple carbs like processed sugar. At the same time, they are very easily stored as fat.

Protein, on the other hand, can undergo a process by which it is turned into sugar — this is called "glycogenesis."

This process takes energy — and so, the "calories" that exist in protein, if it is used for energy, reduces slightly due to the necessary process of converting protein into an energy source. So, protein is an inefficient source of energy, but when it comes to calories, that's a good thing.

This means that the more protein you eat (instead of carbs), the harder your body has to work to turn that food into energy, increasing the caloric cost of digestion.

The double-benefit of eating protein instead of carbs whenever you can is that (1) the caloric cost of digestion raises your TDEE slightly, (2) the caloric value of your food intake decreases slightly, giving you a combined edge on your calorie deficit that carbs don't give you.

3. Carbs can inhibit fat oxidation.

If your body has access to glucose, it will burn glucose, and not fat. Don't let this think that it really matters how many carbs you eat compared to fat. It doesn't.

At the end of each day, your body settles all accounts, and the only thing that really matters is a calorie deficit. However, you can put your body in a "fat burning state" (called "ketosis") — which means your body is burning fat, not glucose, for energy — in which you know for a fact that you are losing body fat as you're exercising.

Just keep in mind is that you can eat zero *carbs*, and be in ketosis for a whole month, and still gain fat if you eat more calories than you consume.

Even if you're in "fat burning mode," if you

overeat, your body will just replace the fat stores
you burned with your excess calories.

Remember: There is no "golden ratio" of carbs
to protein that will cause your fat to instantly
melt away. Cutting calories is one great strategy
to decrease your caloric intake, and nail your
calorie deficit.

35
Can I drink alcohol during my cut?

We hear lots of "health myths" about alcohol:

"A glass of red wine is healthy for your heart."
"A shot of whiskey will clear out your sinuses."
"Racehorses drink Guinness!"

There you go. Free license to drink wine, liquor, and beer for your health! Sadly, these myths simply serve as another cluster of rocks beneath the waves, threatening to smash your willpower into 1,000 pieces.

So, can you drink alcohol during a cut? A little "Yes" and a lot "No."

1. Yes, Drink!

In one sense, drinking alcohol is just another way to ingest calories. Your body will metabolize the liquor with your liver and your brain, so you won't get any immediate "energy" out of them, but rather, those calories will either "intoxicate" you, or be stored as fat in the gut.

Remember when we said that 1g of Carbs = 4 calories, 1g of Protein = 4 calories, and 1g of Fat = 9 calories? Well, 1g of alcohol = 7 calories. And what isn't turned into a neurotoxin turns immediately into fat.

So, here's a calorie guide to your favorite alcohols.

Have fun! Just a little tip: if you're consulting this chart to see which kind of alcohol is the lowest-calorie way to "unwind" from a long day at the office, the answer is: flavorless vodka and diet tonic (tonic water has calories). It'll get you the most neurological bang for the least caloric buck.

Type of Alcohol	Calories

Beer

Light Beer	100 calories, 12 oz.
Belgium Ale	140 calories, 12 oz.
Blue Moon	170 calories, 12 oz.

Wine

Low-Alcohol Red Wine	100 calories, 6 oz.
High-Alcohol Red Wine	190 calories, 6 oz.
Low-Alcohol White Wine	120 calories, 6 oz.
High-alcohol White Wine	210 calories, 6 oz.

Liquor

80 Proof	70 calories, 1 oz.
100 proof	85 calories, 1 oz.

Mixers

Tonic/Club Soda	125 calories, 4 oz.
Soda	50 calories, 4 oz.
Bitters	20 calories, 1 tbsp.
Sugar Cube	10 calories, 1 cube
Lime	20 calories, 1 lime.

2. Just Kidding. Definitely Don't Drink During Your Cut.

A few reasons not to drink during your cut:

1. When you drink, you're more likely to eat.

If you have to choose between a shot of vodka and 3 oz. of chicken, when you're in a calorie deficit, you'll opt for the chicken.

And that chicken will make you feel good — like you made the right choice. But if you choose the vodka, you'll eat the chicken anyway. So don't choose the vodka. Always choose the chicken.

2. Alcohol doesn't give you energy.

It won't power your next run, or motivate you to work harder during your next weight lifting session. In fact, it will promote a sedentary lifestyle. You don't "burn calories" by recovering from alcohol consumption. Quite the opposite.

3. Alcohol inhibits exercise performance.

The day after drinking alcohol, you're groggy, you're unmotivated, you're distracted from your goals. And you may not "feel" it, but you'll be hungrier for fatty foods, and weaker during your workouts.

That means drinking alcohol makes it harder to stick to your diet the next day, and it makes it harder for you to effectively work off the calories you're already having a hard time burning.

THe choice is yours. But don't. So much of diet is about habit. And alcohol consumption simply does not promote habits of self-control and sober self-assessment.

Your calorie deficit will weaken your willpower to begin with. If you struggle at all sticking to your calorie deficit, alcohol is the very worst thing you could consume during your cut.

36
How to eat after a cut.

It would be easy to get the idea that you can do a 12-week cut, and then go back to eating pizza again and you'll have a six pack for the rest of your life! at will lead to deep, deep disappointment.

Especially after all this hard work you've put into getting in shape. How much would it suck to look in the mirror in 6 months, after getting in great shape, and think:

"I look exactly like I did before my cut..."

If you go back to eating the way you did before the cut, you will gain all the weight back. So, should you remain in a 25% calorie deficit for the rest of your life?

No.

You'll starve to death. So, this is what you do: It's called "Reverse Dieting."

After your cut, your metabolism will be very optimized — meaning, it will get the most energy out of the least amount of calories. It has adapted to your deficit.

A lot of people call this "metabolic damage." It shows up in victims, er, contestants of " e Biggest

Loser" who have "damaged metabolisms" and have to eat far less after the show.

The thing about metabolic damage is it's completely reversible if you "Reverse Diet" correctly.

After the last week of your cut, add 5% of your calories back per week — probably carbs. Keep lifting weights. Keep doing cardio.

But, let's say your TDEE (total daily energy expended) is 2,000 calories per day, and your deficit was 1,600 per day. Add 100 calories back this week.

Next week, add another 100 calories back. is process will help your metabolism to heal — it will ease your body out of "metabolic hording," and your body will begin to burn calories more liberally.

Here's where it gets a little tricky. Don't keep adding 100 calories per week forever, or you'll gain all the weight back! Only add 100 calories per week until you're eating what's called "Maintenance Calories."

Your goal is to consume the exact number of

calories that you expend. You still have to count calories. But now that you're not trying to hit a deficit, and you've lost your fat, you can eat a lot more than you could during your cut — with a healed metabolism, and no immediate fat loss desired, you'll aim to eat your TDEE calories exactly.

It's important for you to watch the scale here. It's natural for you to gain a little weight back, as your body will fill with water and glucose when you're not in a calorie deficit. If you find you're starting to gain more than 5 pounds, take 100 calories off for the next week. Adjust, until you find your equilibrium.

When you've successfully "Reverse Dieted" out of your cut, and you can consume your TDEE, you've successfully completed a cut! Congratulations. You've done what few can do — lose the weight, and find a way to *keep it off*. If we were talking in person, I'd buy you an iced green tea from Starbucks and ask you what the hardest part was for you.

Instead, if you complete your cut and want to talk, please email me at theofitco@gmail.com. I'd love to hear your story.

37

How do I keep myself from falling into poor body image during a cut?

This will be a very hard answer to hear. Especially for you soul-searchers out there who want to have their emotions dialed in before they commit to some life-overhaul.

But here's the hard truth:

If you wait to have the right motivations to get in shape, you'll never get in shape. There's no meaningful body transformation without a little body hatred, without a little dysmorphia.

Is it healthy to hate your body? If it gets you a healthy body, then yes — yes it is. Don't let the the ideal of a "healthy body image" sabotage an actually healthy body. You're not anorexic.

Stop eating so much crap. Start exercising a lot more. Those are the eternal, twin laws of fat loss.

38

I'm naturally scrawny— what do I do if I want to gain muscle instead of lose fat?

If you have trouble gaining weight, and you have a natural six-pack but feel "scrawny," then you don't want to do a "cut" — you want to do a "bulk."

Google "Bodybuilding.com bulking plan" and survey the multiple options they have. Most people have trouble eating less to lose fat, but your struggle will be to eat a lot more while you lift a lot more weights.

I'm hoping to come out with a "bulking" book that complements this one, but the weight lifting principles are common to cutting and bulking.

39

How do I look like an Instagram model?

Here's the crazy truth: Most Instagram models are on steroids.

WHAT?!

Yeah, shocker. I didn't realize that until someone told me. en, I did a little research, and it was super obvious.

Ever look at a "Model" on instagram and think, "That guy looks bigger than Superman! How did he get like that?" The answer is Steroids.

Arnold Schwarzenegger took steroids. All the big bodybuilders take steroids. Someone with an unreal amount of veins popping through their abs and has shoulders 4 times the size of his waist — probably on steroids.

Don't compare yourselves to these people. Check out Mike Matthews (muscleforlife.com) — he is a great example of a "natural" (no steroids) lifter who is able to accomplish great fitness goals without steroids.

Don't use steroids. They're so psychologically addicting, most people who begin using them continue to use them for 20 years. Many want to stop using them, but they suppress the human stress hormone (Cortisol), so that when they lift weights, they never feel tired.

Understandably, when you're off steroids, Cortisol can hit you like a ton of bricks. And you can be in withdrawal of that experience for the rest of your life — having the chemical experience of essentially being a god. Not to mention the fact that they're illegal in the U.S., don't take them.

Back to Instagram models:

> They photoshop themselves.
> They take steroids.
> They have special lighting.
> They don't actually look like that ...
> most of them, most of the time.

So don't think you're a fitness failure because you don't look like a skeleton humanoid (who tans). You'd be surprised what a lot of these "models" look like on their days off — it's surprisingly normal.

40

Isn't the goal of "looking good" egotistical?

No. If you like the way a six-pack looks, pursue it. If you don't, then don't. But don't let someone bully you into thinking your fitness goals are narcissistic.

They probably have shame dynamics about their own body, and you expressing your fitness goals stirred up embarrassment in them about their own body.

You do you. Pursue your goals. It's a virtuous thing to change your body. Many times, people who learn to transform their bodies also learn the principles of mental toughness that they need to change every other area of their lives.

Change your body, and you could very well tap into a level of discipline that empowers you to transform the rest of your life.

Part 7

PERS PECT IVE

41

Developing a weight training routine

It's difficult to describe all the workouts you need to learn in order to lift 5 times per week. If you want to get shredded, you really need to work out at least 5 times per week. at doesn't mean you need to do a full weight lifting session with cardio and a cycling class 5 days a week.

But it does mean you need to do at least 45 minutes of intense exercise at least 5 days per week. It's just necessary to achieve the kind of caloric deficit you need in order to see meaningful fat loss.

There are a few places to go to find out how to organize your weight-lifting routine. You can Google "Muscle For Life Develop Workout Plan" or "Bodybuilding.com Develop Workout Plan."

Or, I've developed a full workout plan for every fitness level (and for gym/bodyweight options) with videos for each exercise at https://theo.fit/core.

This sort of routine should add about 750-1000 calories to the TDEE of a 200 pound man, depending on the rigor with which he engages in his exercise.

Essentially, your routine should look something like this:

Day 1	Chest Day
Incline Barbell Bench	10x3
Flat Dumbbell Bench	6x5
Decline Barbell Bench	5x6
Cable Crossover	3x10
Machine Fly	2x15
Push-Ups	1x30
Cardio	30 Minutes
Day 2	Back Day
Deadlift	10x3
Barbell Row	6x5
Dumbbell Row	5x6
Cable Lat Pull-Down	3x10
Cardio	30 Minutes
Day 3	Shoulders Day
Dumbbell Military Press	8x5
Arnold Press	6x10
Side / Front Raise	3x15
Cardio	30 Minutes
Day 4	Cardio Day
Cardio	60 Minutes
Day 5	Arm Day
Barbell Curl + Skull Crusher	3x10
Dumbbell Curl + Tricep Extension	1 Rep/Pound of Weight

Cable Curl + Cable Extension	1 Rep/Pound of Weight
Cardio	30 Minutes
Day 6	**Leg Day**
Back Squat	10x3
Front Squat	6x5
Hip Thruster	5x6
Lunges	3x10
Quad Extension	2x15
Hamstring Curl	1x30
Day 7	**Rest Day**

42

A 4-week calorie deficit tracker

Use the chart on the following pages to track your calorie deficits each day. I recommend using a journal — you can buy (on Amazon) a journal I created for the very principles we've been discussing, called *Finally Fit: Beat Laziness, Get Unstuck, and Finally Make Your Goals Stick*.

Finally Fit is a much more detailed journal. So if you're the kind of person who needs a lot of structure in order to make your diet work, I recommend something like that.

A regular Moleskine journal works as well, if you want to customize your program to your preferences.

But, just to spare you another purchase, I've included a chart for you here. I recommend you don't fill it out in the book, as you might need to start over, or use it again. Simply use it as a template for a blank notebook you already possess, if you so desire.

Day	Weight	TDEE	Consumed	Deficit
4-Week Calorie Deficit Record				
Week 1				
1				
2				
3				
4				
5				
6				
7				
Week 2				
1				
2				
3				
4				
5				
6				
7				
Week 3				
1				
2				
3				
4				
5				

6				
7				
Week 4				
1				
2				
3				
4				
5				
6				
7				

43

Create a "big picture" calorie deficit

So far, we've talked a lot about hitting your daily calorie deficit. And that's extremely important — hitting one day's calorie deficit is as important as taking one step forward in a marathon. But it can also help to have a "macro" perspective on your deficit.

Your goal isn't really to hit a 500 calorie deficit 84 days in a row (12 weeks), right? Let's break down the amount of calories you would need over 12 weeks, how that translates into "overall fat lost," and then how that translates into a daily deficit.

12-Week Deficit Chart		
Fat Loss Goal (In Pounds)	12-Week Calorie Deficit	Daily Deficit Necessary to Meet Goal
10	35,000	
15	52,500	625
20	70,000	833
25	87,500	1,042
30	105,000	1,250

Now, it's probably not healthy to exceed a 1,250 calorie deficit per day. However, somehow, at a 1,000 calorie deficit, I lost about 50 pounds in 3-4 months. So sometimes, with consistency, your body will burn more fat than you expect.

So, if your fat loss goals exceed 30 pounds (even though, with strict adherence, you will likely lose more than that on a 1,250 deficit), here is a chart translating a daily deficit for your goal over a 24-

24-Week Deficit Chart

Fat Loss Goal (In Pounds)	12-Week Calorie Deficit	Daily Deficit Necessary to Meet Goal
35	122,500	729
40	140,000	833
45	157,500	937
50	175,000	1,041
55	192,500	1,146
60	210,000	1,250

week period, extending your "cut" period from 3 months to 6 months. is extension allows you to maintain some sanity, and protect your health (and strength) in a deficit.

MORE RESOURCES:

THEO.FIT

BECOME A PREMIUM MEMBER:

THEO.FIT/MEMBERSHIP

THEO.FIT